Natural Cures for Acne

Eliminate Pimples Naturally

By M. Usman

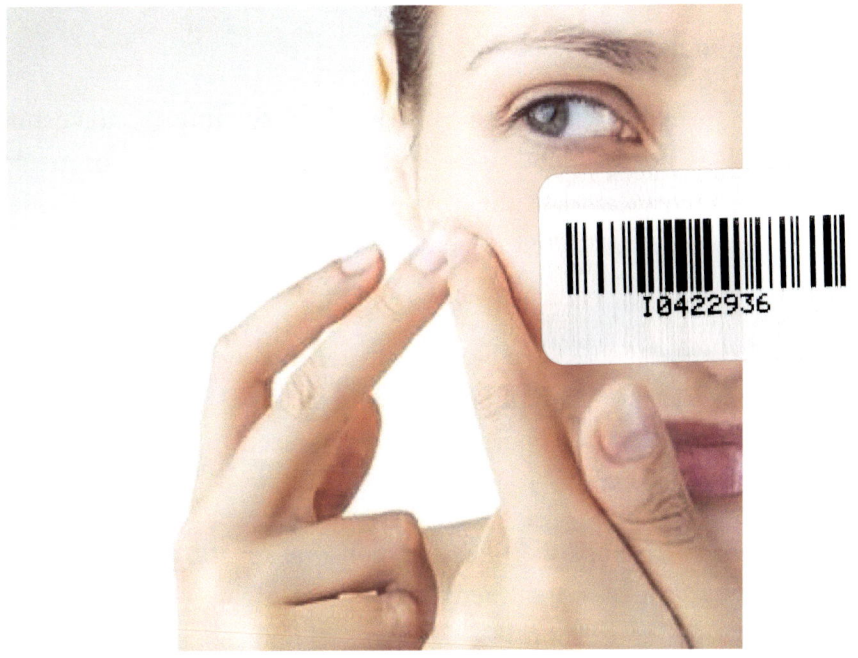

Health Learning Series

Mendon Cottage Books

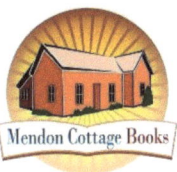

JD-Biz Publishing

Disclaimer

The information is this book is provided for informational purposes only. It is not intended to be used and medical advice or a substitute for proper medical treatment by a qualified health care provider. The information is believed to be accurate as presented based on research by the author.

The contents have not been evaluated by the U.S. Food and Drug Administration or any other Government or Health Organization and the contents in this book are not to be used to treat cure or prevent disease or mental illness.

The author or publisher is not responsible for the use or safety of any diet, procedure or treatment mentioned in this book. The author or publisher is not responsible for errors or omissions that may exist.

Warning

The Book is for informational purposes only and before taking on any diet, treatment or medical procedure it is recommended to consult with your primary care provider.

Our books are available at

1. Amazon.com
2. Barnes and Noble
3. Itunes
4. Kobo
5. Smashwords
6. Google Play Books

Table of Contents

Introduction

How badly we all wanted to be a teenager when we were little kids? But who knew this teenage comes with incalculable challenges of acne. Being a teenager, you have gone through the times, when you looked at yourself in the mirror and screeched, "No, not again, a pimple". Then surely there is rush to peel your face in order to make this bad mark disappear. If so, then we are here to help you out.

If you are an acne sufferer, then this book will help you find out quick and easy recipes to kick the pimple out of your skin. On reading this book, you will have a new understanding of your problem. Each chapter of this book contains all the information that can help you to combat acne and give yourself a fresh morning.

SECTION # 1: A Glance At Acne

Chapter # 1: Acne: An Introduction

Acne is a common skin disease. It is characterized by blocked hair follicles with greasy secretions from oil producing glands. Acne lesions are most commonly referred as pimples. Debris and bacteria can accumulate in these clogged pores. This can lead to inflammation. It causes blemishes to develop on skin. It can take various forms including blackheads, whiteheads and papules.

A painful acne bump doesn't appear suddenly overnight. It takes two or more weeks. In this period the causes of acne are hard at work to bring out the ugly looking pimple.

These lesions are mostly common on face, but they can also occur on the neck, back, shoulders, upper arms and chest. The reason behind this is that oil producing glands are abundant in these areas. The symptoms of acne can be mild, moderate or severe. In cases of severe cases, scarring can develop.

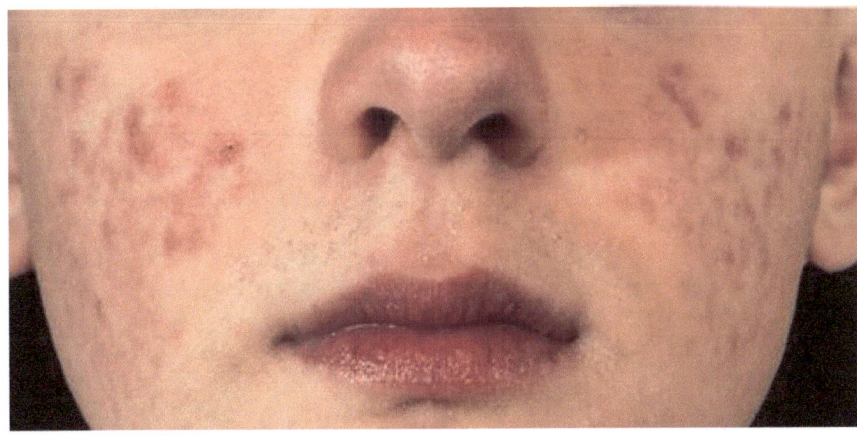

Chapter # 2: Understanding Pimples

Skin of human is a beautiful gift of nature. Beauty is surely in the eyes of viewer but in reality, one has to be beautiful to be praised. Clear skin is another blessing of God. As skin is the most sensitive part of the body, it gets easily attacked by the pollution and dirt in the air.

Human skin has many pores containing oil. These pores contain oily glands. These glands produce sebum, which is an oily secretion containing dead skin cells. It carries these dead cells through the follicles to the surface of skin. When these follicles get blocked due to any reason, oil accumulates under the skin. The result of which is the growth of pimple. This plug can get infected with a pus forming bacterium called *Propionibacteium acnes* that normally inhabit the skin. Plugged follicles with greasy material cause these bacteria to grow tremendously.

Formation of Skin Pimples and Acnes

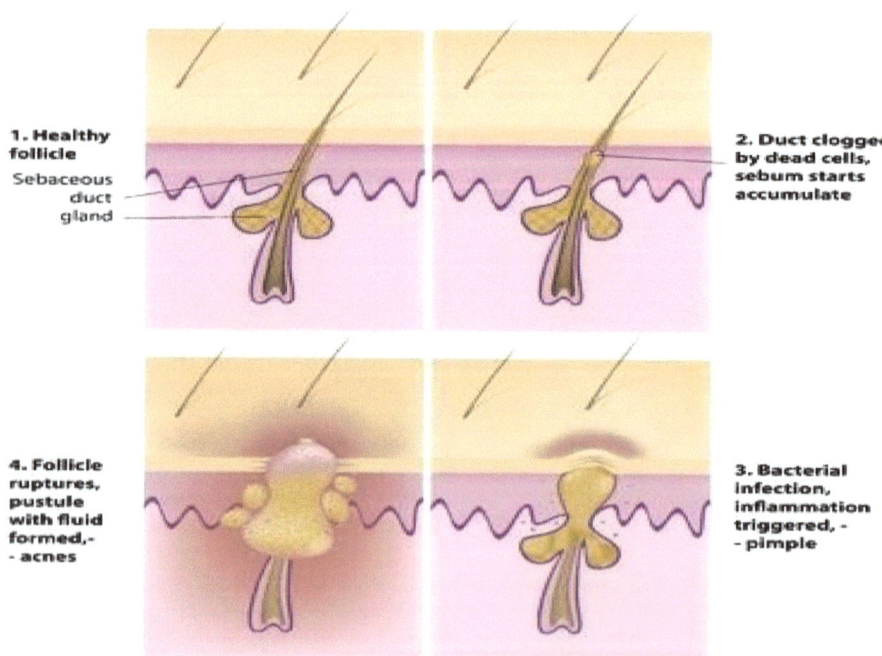

1. **Healthy follicle**
Sebaceous duct gland

2. **Duct clogged by dead cells, sebum starts accumulate**

4. **Follicle ruptures, pustule with fluid formed, - acnes**

3. **Bacterial infection, inflammation triggered, - pimple**

Acne can progress in following manners:

- When hair follicle is incompletely blocked, it results in blackhead
     formation.
- When hair follicle is completely blocked, it results in whitehead formation.
- When acne is superficial, it appears as pimple without pus.
- When pimple pushes down into skin, it results into a sac containing pus.

Chapter # 3:Time To Worry

Anyone can get acne. But it is a curse of adolescence. Most of the acne sufferers are teenagers. Adults and even babies can get awful acne.

Acne commonly starts during puberty between the ages of 10 to 13 years and tends to be worse in people with oily skin. Girls are more prone to acne than boys. Most acne cases in girls occur between 14 to 17 years of age. In boys, acne pops out between the age of 16 to 19 years.

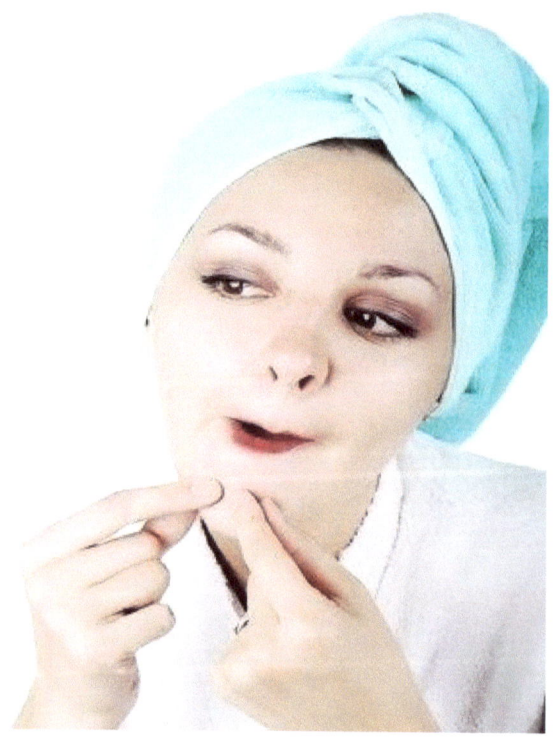

Most people get rid of acne by the time they reach their 30's. But some people having sensitive skin bear acne even in their 50's. Most people experience repeated outburst for several years. The symptoms of acne start to improve as the sufferer grows older.

Chapter # 4: Recipe Card of Acne

"Acne is a complex medical condition caused by four factors: hormones, inflammation, bacteria, and dead skin cells that clog pores," says dermatologist Jessica Krant, founder of the Art of Dermatology.

Any one of these factors can attack you from anywhere. Therefore be alarmed of the following causes of acne:

- Overproduction of sebum:

The primary cause of acne in teenagers is an increase in the level of androgens. This increment in hormone levels enhances oil production, which in turn kicks sebum production into overdrive. The fluctuating hormone levels in women can also occur in following conditions:

- During menstrual cycle.
- During pregnancy and menopause.
- While the use of birth control pills.

Medication:

Several hormonal medications can worsen acne:

Steroids are well known for causing acne and pimples. The common steroids, used to treat lung diseases, spark off oil producing gland. This steps-up the breakout and blemishes.

Contraceptive agents can sometimes aggravate acne in females. These agents contain progesterone or estrogen, which can lead to hormonal imbalance in the body.

Bacteria:

Bacteria can grow exponentially in the greasy environment of plugged follicles. It leads to inflammation and formation of blackheads.

Diet:

A study completed by the Australia's RMIT University and Royal Melbourne Hospital Department of Dermatology made found out that certain carbohydrates affect acne development. Researchers believe that carbohydrate-rich food e.g. potato chips, bread etc., can actuate the acne. These food products can cause glucose and insulin to peak affecting development and severity of acne.

Chemicals:

Cleansing with harsh chemicals can irritate the skin and can cause acne. Some soaps and face washes contain dangerous chemicals that can cause acne to flourish.

Allergens:

Any allergen such as gluten, dairy and eggs may be responsible for acne. Some people develop acne due to allergy to meat products.

Irritation:

Skin may also get irritated with friction from tight collars or helmets. This also can cause acne.

Family history:

Some people may have genetic predisposition to develop acne. Such people are more prone to skin problems.

Chapter # 5: What Makes Acne Grow Enormously?

All of a sudden, you have a zit to numerous red spots on your skin. You wonder, what went so wrong that this happened. So you blame your ignorance for all this or even that pretty new shade of eyeliner you've been wearing. Triggers of this distressing condition might be poor sleep, dairy diet or mental stress.   These factors are the hidden culprits that make you meet this outbreak. Be alert to these often-sneaky causes of acne.

Mental stress:

The average acne sufferer's skin contains clogged pores that they can't even appreciate. Stress produces an inflammatory response in the body that can cause these pores to break their walls off. When this happens, the body shows redness around the broken pore and a zit appears. Stress also makes the hormones such as adrenalin, to get out of their cages. Higher androgen levels can also lead to more acne.

Menstrual cycle:

It seems to happen every month that your skin appears to be clearing up nicely. Suddenly acne starts bashing in your face. It is just around the time of menstruation. It is a scientifically proven fact that acne sufferers' menstrual cycle directly impacts their acne. There are hormonal changes and fluctuations that happen in a women's cycle. These peaking hormones (mainly androgens) cause the increase in facial oily glands. This excess oil starts filling up the facial pores and causes acne.

Hot climate:

Do you think weather can work with acne? If yes then you are right. Any kind of change in weather and humidity does affect skin for better or worse depending on skin type. Oily skin in hot and humid climate provide favorable environment for the bacteria to grow and develop acne. Moreover, hot weather pushes more oil out of its pockets.

Makeup:

Many makeup artists will tell you that makeup should be used to enhance your facial features. That's easy to say when you have a clear facial canvas. But for others facing acne trouble, makeup may seem like the only cure to hide the flaws. Unfortunately, it does not happen in reality. All the makeup products containing oil can throw you more towards the hell of acne. Oil prone areas such as the forehead, nose or chin are particularly vulnerable especially when excess makeup is used to cover them.

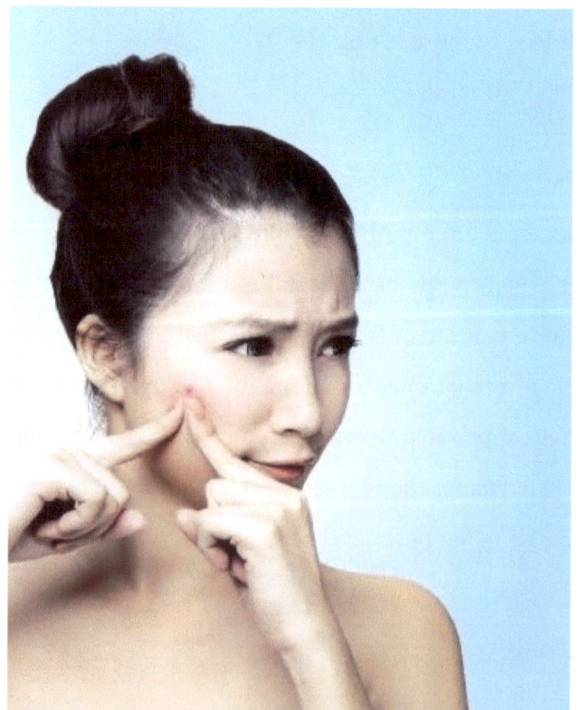

Tweaking the pimple:

If you are in hurry to get rid of a pimple, don't squeeze it. Squeezing a pimple is more in favor to worsen the condition. It can also leave a permanent scar mark.

Bad hygiene:

Bad hygiene is a culprit behind the worsening of acne. People, who are not in the habit of washing off (mainly their face) after coming back home, are more likely to develop acne. Pollutants on your face, if not washed properly, can provide the basis for zits.

SECTION # 2: Give a Punch to Acne

As it is said earlier, acne is a common problem now days. It is an awful reality in the life of teenagers and adults. It leaves behind the scars and makes skin dull and patchy. Acne sufferers often feel dejected due to these unsightly scar marks. They make every possible effort to get rid of this and spend a lot of their time and money rushing to the dermatologists and on buying expensive skin products. These products often contain harmful chemicals which instead of curing can exaggerate the condition.

Fortunately nature has blessed us with many useful things. As nature has a cure for every disease, acne can also be cured by using natural products. The only thing you have to do is bolt from your seat and rush towards the kitchen, the place having solution for your problem.

When a pimple rears its ugly red head, following simple natural remedies can help to wipe it out. Following chapters cover the most beneficial natural cure for acne.

Sanative lifestyle
Barge in your kitchen
Hunt for herbs
Diet for right

Chapter # 6: Sanative Lifestyle

Your health depicts your lifestyle and your face shows how you treat your body. A little concern towards your routine can do magic. Following points can be helpful for the basic skin care:

A healthy start:

Always give a kicking start to your day with a healthy and nutritious breakfast. It will pack an encouraging energy punch to see your whole day.

Dabble in water:

The habit of drinking plenty of water can do wonders. Your body needs to get rid of all the waste material produced during metabolism. Water cleanses your body and takes away all the toxicity. Washing your face frequently refreshes your skin. It removes the dirt and doesn't let the pimple pop out.

Never skip a meal:

Skipping meals can cause blood glucose to rise. This rise can lead to significant hormonal changes in the body including insulin and glucocorticoids. And then you end up having acne with this hormonal turbulence. But it doesn't mean you've to stuff your plate with anything you get your hands on. Eat healthy, this is explained in detail in the subsequent chapter.

Look before use:

Now days the use of face wash and facial scrubs has increased. Excessive use of these chemical containing products can irritate the skin worsening acne.

Don't pinch:

Squeezing or pinching a pimple can cause scarring. If you press a pimple with contaminated hand, it produces blemishes. Don't squeeze it. Let it settle down itself.

What touches your face:

Avoid resting your hands and objects, such as pen, on your face. It can grime your face. Keep your hair off your face. Caps can also pose the problem, if you are sweating. Sweat, oil and dirt can cause acne.

Get more sleep:

Sleep relaxes your mind. It reduces the physiological stress. After having enough sleep, you feel fresh. Your freshness is always there on your skin. Moreover, sleep decrease the level of stress hormones. The role of stress hormones in the development of acne has been explained previously.

Be gentle to sugar:

A study published in the *American journal of Nutrition* found that people who consumed a diet less in sugar had fewer breakouts of acne. Certain food cause increased blood glucose. This can lead to hormonal changes and acne. So go easy on sugar rich products, sodas, bakery products and fast food.

Grasp fresh air:

Air containing oxygen is a blessing for your skin. Make it a habit to do regular exercise in fresh air. It improves your blood circulation. Hence it increases oxygen supply to skin, helping cell renewal.

Cover the sun:

When you are in sun, it dries out your skin and makes it burn. It can cause dehydration and provide more chances of clogged pores. Therefore make it a habit to wear sun protection whenever you are sun-kissed.

Chapter # 7: Intrude On Your Kitchen

For you, your kitchen is a place where you can cook. But for us, it is a drug store for your problem. Solution to your pressure points is in your closed cabinets. Now open your cabinets and get your recipe ingredients. All the following simple ingredients can do a splendid job. Here is the recipe card for curing your acne problem:

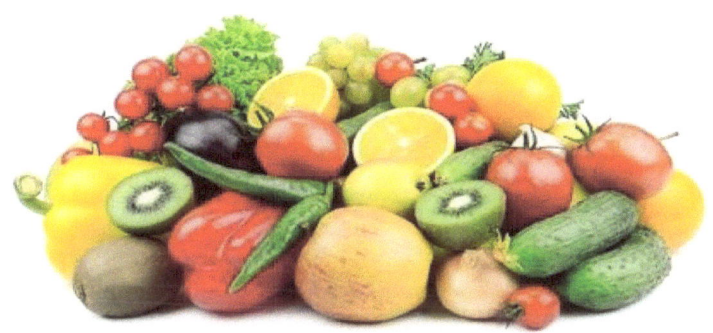

Sprinkle the Baking soda:

For baking lovers, baking soda must be there in their recipe card. But for acne sufferers, it must be on their face. This is an absolute favorite natural remedy for acne. Baking soda helps to reduce inflammation. It exfoliates and helps to remove dead skin cells. It does wonders to old scars or acne marks.

How to use:

Take a few teaspoons of baking soda and mix it with warm water until it forms a paste. Apply the paste to the affected areas. Leave it on for 10 to 15 minutes. It will get dry. Rub it for one minute, then rinse. It will remove dead skin and will aid in cellular renewal.

Grate Cucumber:

Cucumber is a basic element of your salads. The water content of cucumber keeps you hydrated in sun peaked days. It also has variety of benefits for your skin. It is a natural astringent that cleanses the pores on your face. It does so by removing oil and dirt from the pores.

How to use:

You can use cucumber slices directly onto your face. It helps to soothe the skin.

Take out juice of a cucumber. Apply this on the affected area using cotton ball. Leave it to dry for few minutes, and then rinse it off. To make the marks disappear, apply it every day. It gives your skin a fresh look.

Use cucumber as facial mask. Make thin paste of it with half cup of yogurt and apply it. Leave it for 30 minutes then wipe it off. It moisturizes your skin. Regular use of this mask keeps you free from acne.

You can also use cucumber juice by mixing it with equal quantity of rose water and coconut water. It will clear your skin with a glow.

Play with Tomato:

Tomato is a main ingredient of your recipes including steaks and salads. Now treat this part of your food as your make over. Tomato has vitamin A, C and K, and also lycopene. These essentials can be found in any acne treating creams. Tomatoes help keeping acne dry.

How to use:

Treat your face gently with a slice of fresh tomato. Rub this slice on the affected area.

You can also simply mash a tomato to pulp form. This pulp can be applied as facial mask. With regular application, you'll see the difference.

Mash the Potato:

Till now, you have used potatoes for making fries and pudding. But now you will learn how to use it to enhance your beauty. Potato is rich in vitamin C and B. It also contains niacin. Vitamin C helps in collagen production, which helps to heal the damage of your skin. Vitamin B is responsible for regeneration of skin cells. Niacin helps to lighten the hyper-pigmented areas.

How to use:

Take a potato from your pantry. Cut it into two halves. Rub one half on the problematic area. It will not only treat acne but also helps to lighten the skin.

Squeeze the Lemon:

You may have used lemon for multiple times in variety of foods. Now take another journey with this small but potent element of cure. Lemon juice is the most beneficial cure for acne scars. It helps to minimize the discoloration.

Vitamin C content of lemon helps to keep the skin fresh and glowing. Lemon also contains antioxidants. These antioxidants help to keep the damaging free radicals away from skin. This makes lemon juice an excellent remedy for pimples.

How to use:

Squeeze a freshly-cut lemon. Dab a little of its juice directly on the affected area. You can apply it using a cotton ball. Leave it overnight and sleep with the thought of clear skin in the morning. Repeat this remedy daily. Regular use will amaze you. But remember that if you've a sensitive skin then never apply it directly to your skin. Dilute it with rose water and apply it then.

Beat the Yoghurt:

You must love sweet yoghurt in the burning season of sun. Now put the can open for your acne. Yoghurt contains vitamins and minerals. These help to increase the immune system and nourish the skin.

How to use:

Use yoghurt as cleanser using cotton.

You can apply it directly on the face.

You can also use yoghurt with a pinch of turmeric. Apply the mixture and let it dry. Rinse with cold water and feel the wonders of yoghurt.

Try the Oatmeal:

Oatmeal is effective for the prevention of acne. It sucks the excess oil from the skin and helps to keep the skin oil free. This prevents the follicles to be clogged with oil.

How to use:

Mix the oatmeal with water. Make a thin paste of it. Apply this mask on your face and wait until it dries. Wipe it off and feel the difference. Regular use can keep the skin away from pimples.

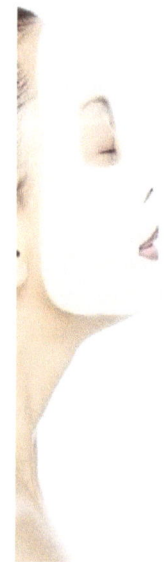

Whip up Whites:

Egg whites are not only to make omelets and mayonnaise. But these make a great natural remedy when used as a facial mask. Egg whites lower the oil production. These also minimize acne by drawing impurities out of pores.

How to use:

To use it, separate the egg white from the yolk. Use a cotton ball to apply this egg white on your face. You can also use your fingers. After few minutes, it will start to tighten up your skin. Leave it for 10 minutes. Rinse it off and feel the difference afterwards.

Be Friends with Garlic:

You may not like garlic when it comes to consuming, give thanks to garlic breath. But just before you discount it completely; let me tell you a fact. Garlic is one of those elements that have been valued for centuries for treating skin problems. Garlic is blessed with antibacterial and antifungal properties and it can cure inflammation too. To expel acne out of your face, you can use garlic.

How to use:

Take a clove of garlic and make thin slices of it. Rub the slices on your skin, particularly the problematic part. Make sure that juice of garlic is applied. Leave it for 15 minutes and rinse.

Take 6 cloves of garlic. Crush them completely and mix with a spoonful of honey and a dash of turmeric powder. Apply this paste directly onto acne with your fingers. Leave it for 15-20 minutes. Rinse with warm water. You can feel the magic of garlic with regular use.

Slam Apple Cider Vinegar on Face:

Apple cider vinegar is a fireball when it comes to act as an acne remedy. It destroys the bacteria that may be causing all the trouble. It also balances the pH of your skin, making trouble for the bacteria to thrive. It is an astringent, like lemon juice and will help to dry up excess oil. Keeping that in mind, don't overdo otherwise it will dry out your skin too much.

How to use:

Wash your face with water and pat dry. Use 1 part vinegar to 3 parts of water. Dip a cotton ball into vinegar and apply it directly to the blemishes. Leave on for at least 10 minutes or overnight. Reapply several times a day. Use a moisturizer afterwards if you feel like your skin is getting dry. Make sure to use apple cider vinegar that is raw and unfiltered. It has the most ingredients.

Flesh a Papaya:

Papaya is an essential ingredient to be used as meat tenderizer. In addition to this, it is also used in a lot of beauty products in the market today. But there is no need to go out of your way to gain its benefits. Plain raw papaya is one of the most beneficial acne remedies. It removes dead skin cells and excess oil from the surface of the skin, leaving it soft and smooth. It also helps to prevent the pus formation.

How to use:

Rinse your face with water and pat dry. Mash up the flesh of the papaya until it is of a consistency that can be easily applied to your skin. Leave it for 15-20 minutes and then rinse it off with warm water.

Slip on a Banana:

Bananas are healthy source of beauty boosting vitamin A, C and E. It moisturizes the skin by giving enough hydration to your skin. Their peels contain an extremely powerful antioxidant that reduces inflammation and encourages healthy cell growth.

How to use:

Try a shine reducing mask by mixing banana with lemon juice. Lemon juice will cut the oil out of pimples. Banana will help to prevent further production of excess oil.

Mash a banana peel and make a paste of it. Rub it on your face in circular motion. When you feel it has covered your face, leave it for 15-30 minutes. Then rinse it off with warm water.

Go for Strawberries:

Strawberries make a home remedy with honey. This combination is widely used in facial scrubs and cleansers. Strawberries encourage the skin to shed off its dead cells. It removes debris and help opening the clogged pores. It also neutralizes the bacteria. It shrinks up the pores a little bit. This prevents production of blocked pores in future and enhances new cell growth.

How to use:

Rinse 3 strawberries and mash them up well. Add 2 teaspoons of honey to this and blend them together thoroughly. Apply it to your face and let the mixture to sit for 20 minutes. Rinse off completely with warm water and pat dry. Use this mixture twice a week for apparent results.'

Give a Try to Orange Peel:

Oranges are refreshing for our taste buds. Our skin needs this freshness too. Acne caused by impurities can be cured with an orange peel mask. Vitamin C in the peel of orange gives the skin an overall good condition. It also acts as astringent which helps to shrink pores.

How to use:

Take a fresh orange and peel it off. Now grind this peel. Add little water to make a thin paste. As right consistency is gained, apply it on your face. Give it 20-30 minutes. Then rinse it off.

Be Sweet to Honey:

Honey not only helps scar tissue to reconstruct, but it also boosts collagen production and softens skin. It also eliminates bacteria growth and inflammation. It gives even skin tone and balances skin pH.

How to use:

Take some honey out of the jar. Apply it all over your face like a mask. Being thick, it helps to dampen the skin. You can apply it with wet hands to make it spread better. Leave it for 10-15 minutes and then wash it off.

Chapter # 8: Hunt For Herbs/Spices

On reading this heading, a question may strike your mind. Why to go for herbs when there are new and advance treatments available in the market? Here lies the answer, it's better to use simple proven and long lasting treatment instead of complex and expensive ones. The effects of drugs and creams last only till the time you use them. Once you'll skip them, acne will catch you again. It not only suppresses the symptoms, but also deals with the disease from deep within, when you treat it with herbal products. This makes herbal treatment an effective one.

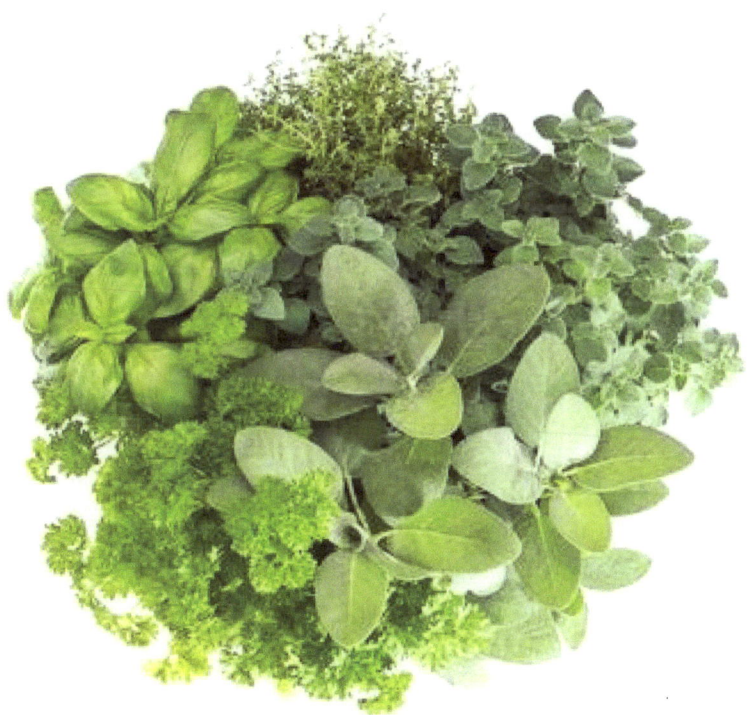

Following herbal remedies that you will come across after reading this chapter, will blow your mind.

Crush Cinnamon:

Cinnamon is a common spice and a flavoring agent. It has anti-microbial properties. You can use cinnamon mixture with honey.

How to use:

Use approximately ½ tablespoon of cinnamon powder and add it to honey. Mix it well to make a paste. Apply this paste on acne and leave overnight. Wash off with lukewarm water the next morning.

Spice it Up With Turmeric:

No wonder that women have always been using turmeric powder to make their skin healthier and glowing. Turmeric made into paste can destroy the inflammation causing bacteria. Turmeric possesses anti-oxidant and anti-inflammatory properties, both of which are helpful to cure acne.

How to use:

You can make a paste of turmeric with milk by mixing 2 tablespoon of turmeric powder with 1 tablespoon of milk. Use your fingers and apply this paste to dry skin. Massage for 10 minutes. The turmeric paste will get dry and will become stiff like mask. Rinse it with water.

You can also use turmeric powder with yoghurt. Take 2 teaspoon of yoghurt and ½ teaspoon of turmeric powder. Make a thin paste and apply it to acne prone skin.

Turmeric can give yellow tinge to skin. To remove this, clean your face with wet cotton.

Latch on the Neem:

We are surrounded by many wonderful things gifted to us by nature, but we don't even know them. Neem is one of such incredible blessings. Neem has an almost magical effect on acne. All your skin problems can be cured by using neem regularly. But the key to this is to use it correctly.

How to use:

Take some fresh neem leaves. Wash them and grind them to make a thin paste. Add turmeric powder to this and apply for 20 minutes. Wash off with cold water. If you don't have fresh leaves, you can use dry leaves powder with water.

Neem leaves paste can also be used with few drops of lemon juice. It is beneficial for oily skin to remove excess oil.

Take Teeny-Weeny Tea Tree Oil:

Tea tree oil is a popular home remedy for acne. It is an essential oil, which can kill skin-dwelling bacteria that cause inflammation.

How to use:

Dilute a few drops of tea tree oil with water. Apply it to skin once or twice a day with a cotton swab. Be careful, not to overuse it. Tea tree oil can dry out your skin, shifting your body to overproduction of oil thus causing acne.

Feel Fresh With Aloe Vera:

The benefits of Aloe Vera are well known all across the world. It is used in moisturizers, lotions and creams in market because of its curative and moisturizing properties. It also lightens skin pigmentation.

How to use:

For treating acne and scars with aloe, wash your face. Apply this gel on face and neck. Leave it for night and wash the next morning.

This gel can also be used as a facial mask. Mix Aloe Vera gel, honey and rose water to make a fine paste and apply this mask on the acne prone areas and wash it off after 20 minutes. A pinch of turmeric to this facial mask can also be added to brighten your complexion.

Chapter # 9: Diet For Right

It is true that what you eat has influence on the way you look. You can keep your skin looking at it its best by having healthy and nutrient-rich diet. Although the thought is still out if oily foods actually cause acne breakouts, it is always good advice to make right food choices and follow a balanced diet. Fruits and vegetables make our skin to glow with all the vitamins and nutrients.

Buff Omega-3 Fatty Acids:

Walnuts, avocados and salmons are rich in omega-3 fatty acids. Add these foods to your diet. It will control sebum production and thus inflammation. Controlling acne is one of the never ending benefits of omega-3 fatty acids.

Take on vitamins:

Vitamin E and C are the most beneficial vitamins for the skin. These are the anti-oxidants and have calming effect. Oranges, grape fruits, lemon, papaya and tomatoes are the rich source of vitamin C. vitamin E can be obtained from green leafy vegetables, olive oil, nuts and sweet potatoes.

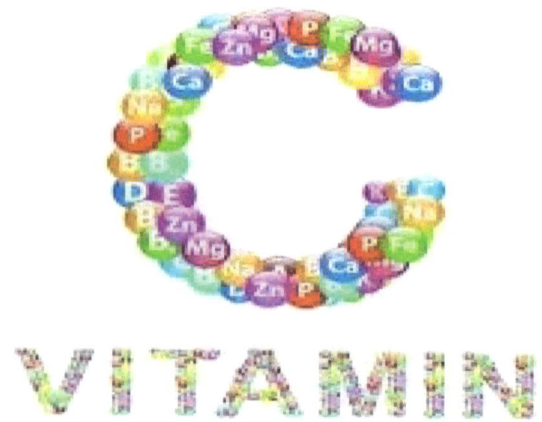

Give Zinc to Vegetarians:

Meat and poultry provide the majority of zinc. Zinc helps to reduce inflammation, promote wound healing. It maintains skin integrity and may reduce skin oil production. Studies show that low blood zinc levels make your skin prone to acne. Therefore vegetarians should take care of their zinc ingestion. But don't go nuts on consuming meat. It would be better to consume white meat instead or red one.

Dodge the sugar:

An emerging body of evidence suggests that eating a diet rich in high glycemic index may be bound to acne breakout. It includes white bread, white rice, pasta, baked goods and anything processed. Excess sugar in the blood causes the body to secrete hormones. These hormones work hard to bring the blood sugar level down. Excess of these hormones make our glands to produce a heap of sebum causing acne. Therefore cut down your sugar intake to keep your body away from acne.

Chapter #10: Preventions

Prevention is always better than cure. Although there is no certain method to prevent acne, there are number of ways to reduce your breakouts. You can prevent your acne breakouts by minor changes in your lifestyle and with little care. Following basic skin care regime is your key to wash out acne.

Do not let your body get dehydrated. Take plenty of water to stay well hydrated.

Exercising daily will not only help you look and feel better but it will also help reduce the frequency of your breakouts. Physical exercise increases the blood flow through the body which will keep your skin looking healthy and radiant.

It is important to wash pillow cases and towels regularly. Dirty stuff can cause pus forming bacteria to thrive.

Acne prone skin needs moisturizing and cleansing. Choose a light and water-based moisturizer to keep your skin hydrant.

Remove makeup before going to bed. Layer of makeup will block the pores of skin and will not let them take a breath. This will end up in acne breakout.

Wash your face only twice a day. Washing removes excess oil and dirt from the skin. But too much washing can irritate the skin.
Use only oil-free skin and hair products. Use makeup that is water-based or labeled as "non-comedogenic".

Reduce stress and relax. Staying calm and happy help to control breakouts

Quit smoking and alcohol consumption. This disturbs the metabolic system of the body. It also dehydrates the skin, making it more prone to acne.

Author Bio

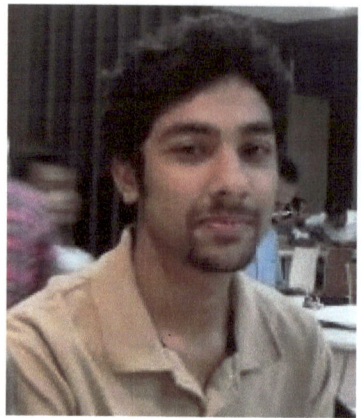

Muhammad Usman is a distinguished medical graduate of Allama iqbal medical college (AIMC). He is a professional writer who has been in the field for more than 4 years. During this time he has produced 10,000+ articles, blogs and eBooks on various niches related to diseases, health, fitness, nutrition and well-being. He is a regular contributor to several journals related to medicine and surgery. He is the editor of several journals and newspapers.

Check out some of the other JD-Biz Publishing books

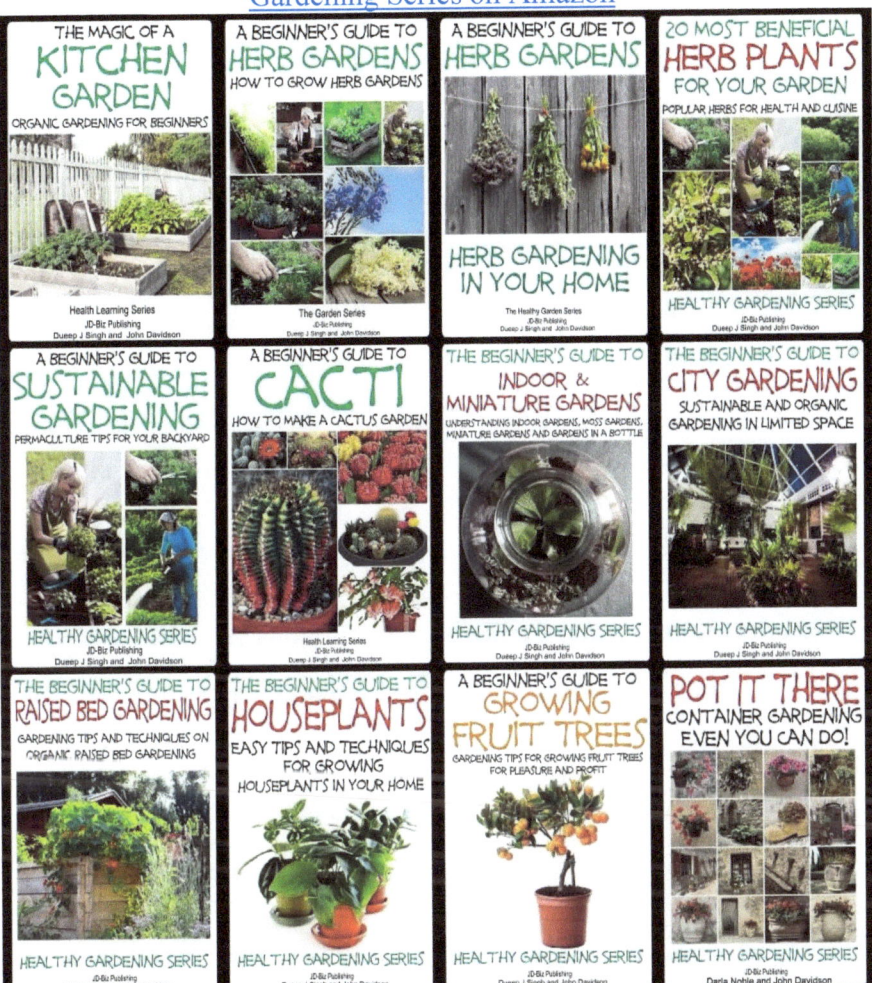

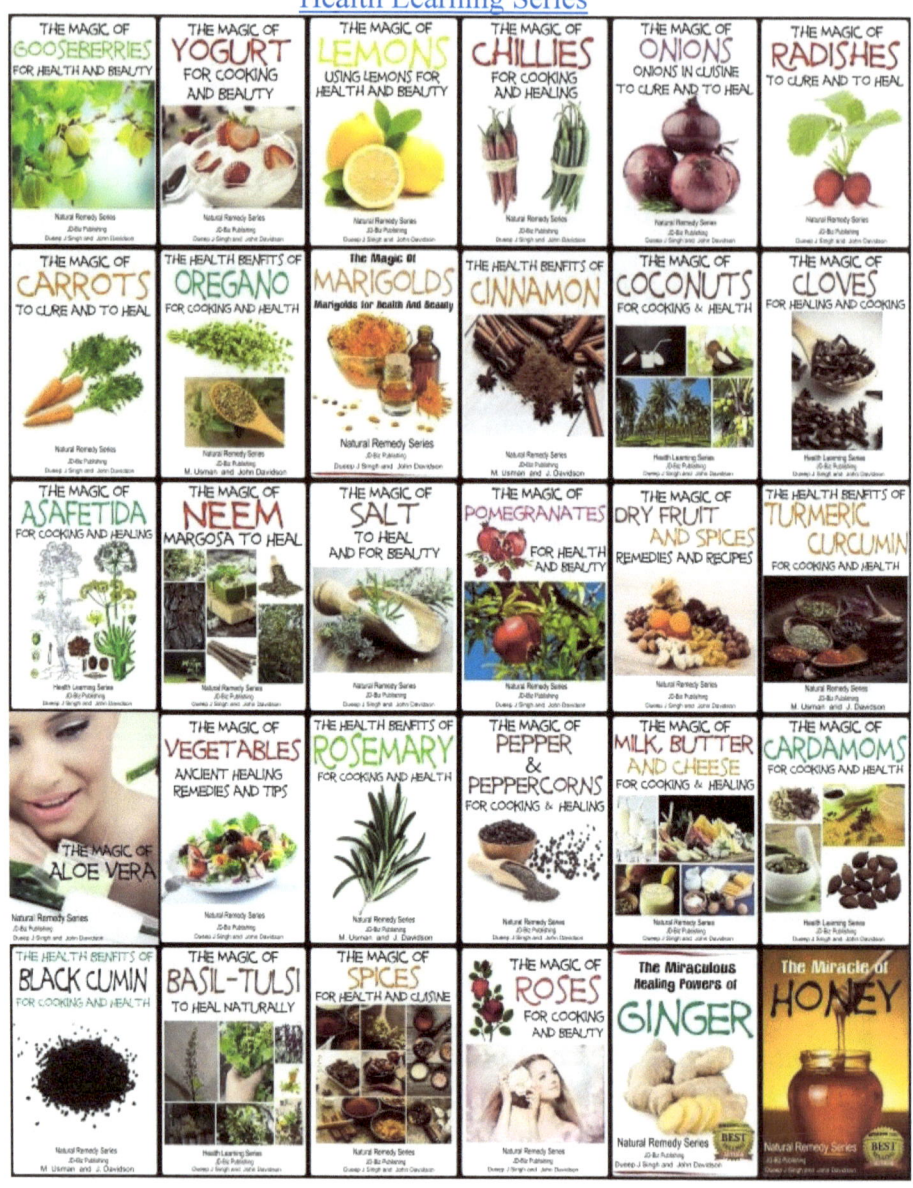

Country Life Books

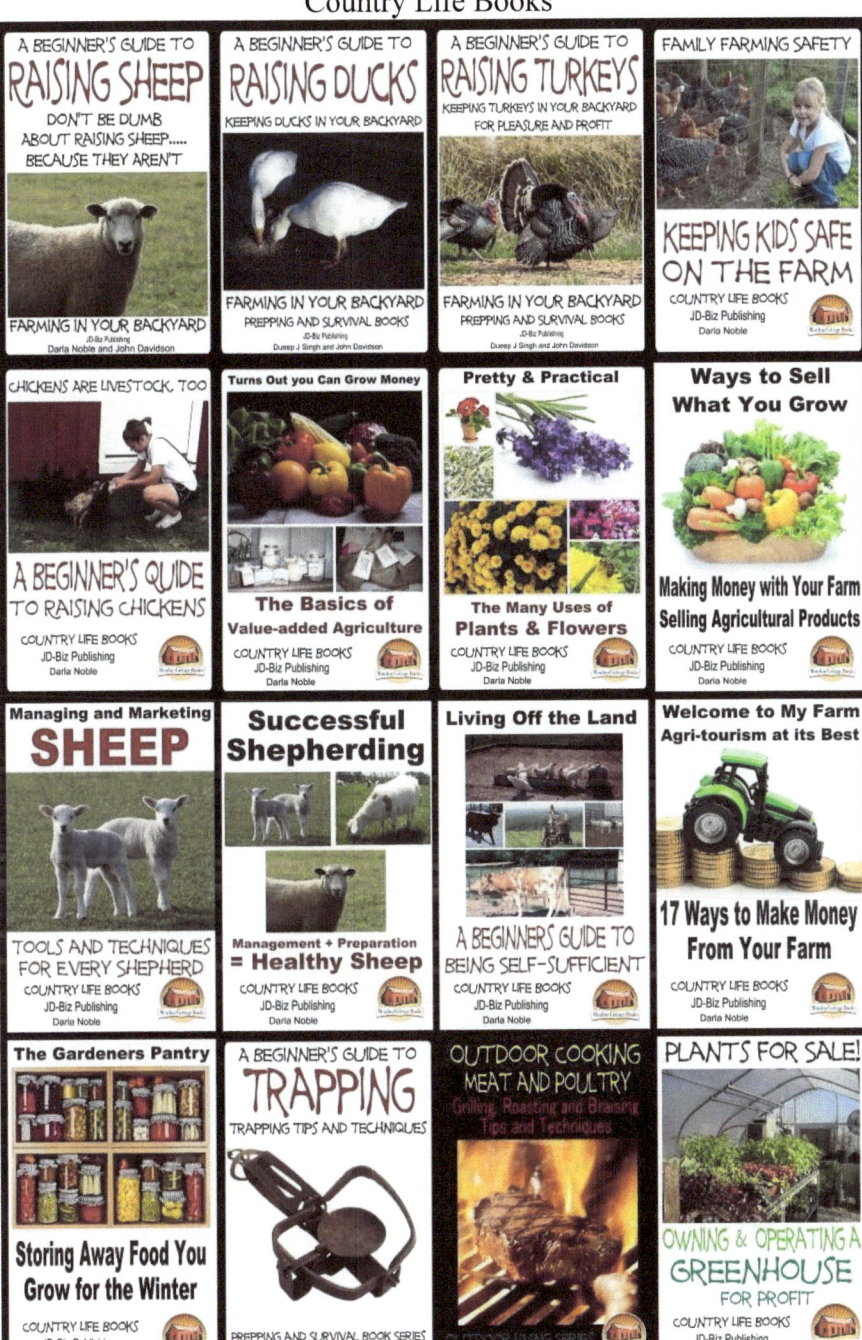

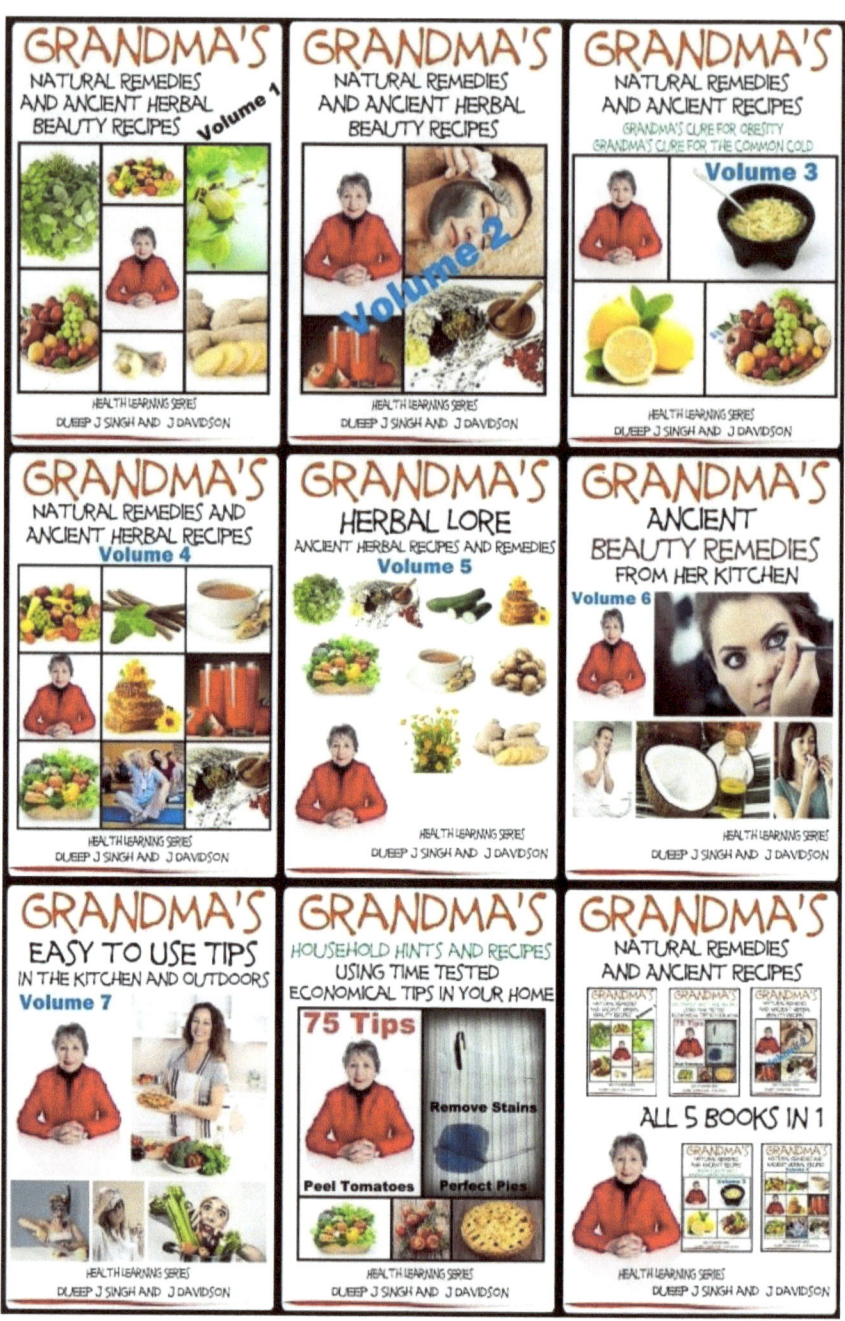

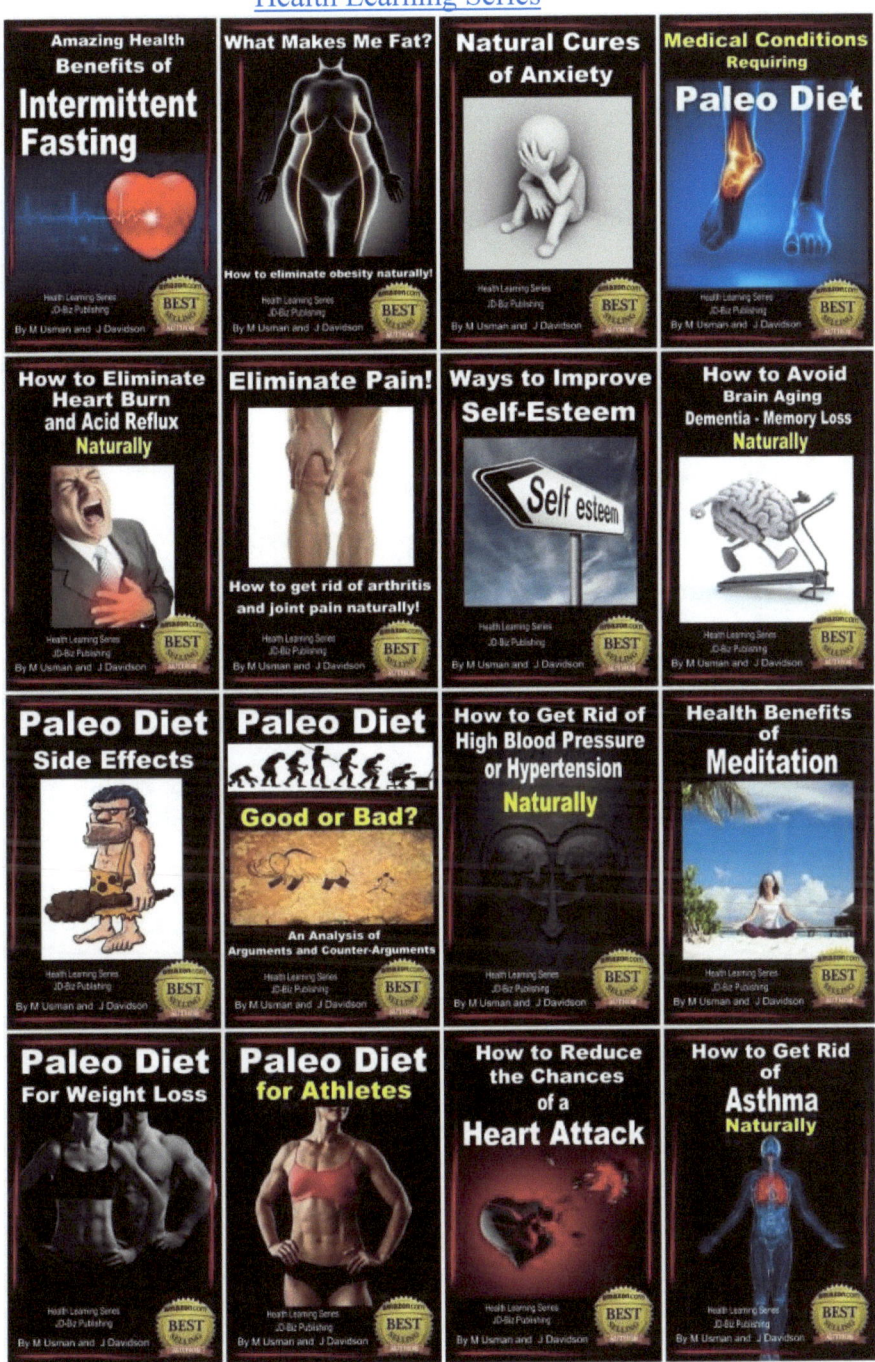

Amazing Animal Book Series

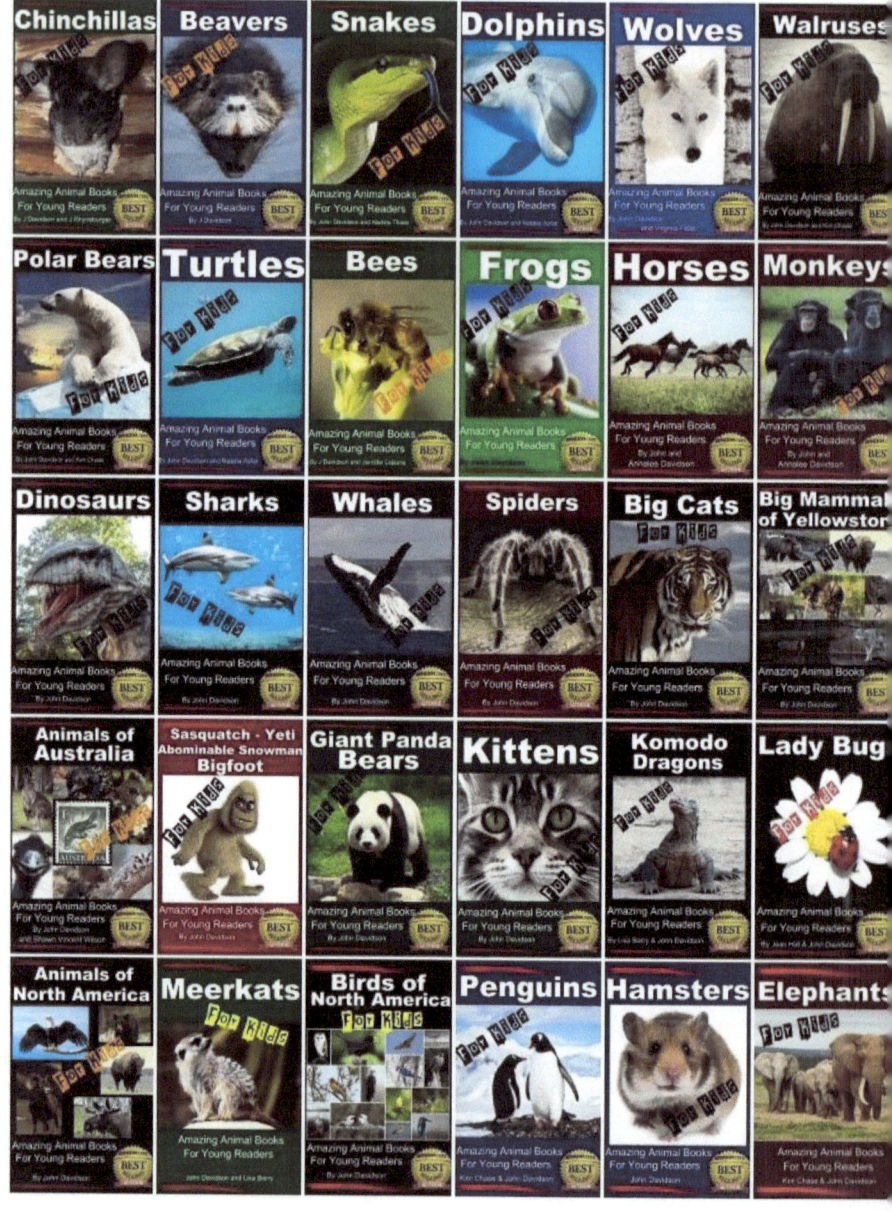

Learn To Draw Series

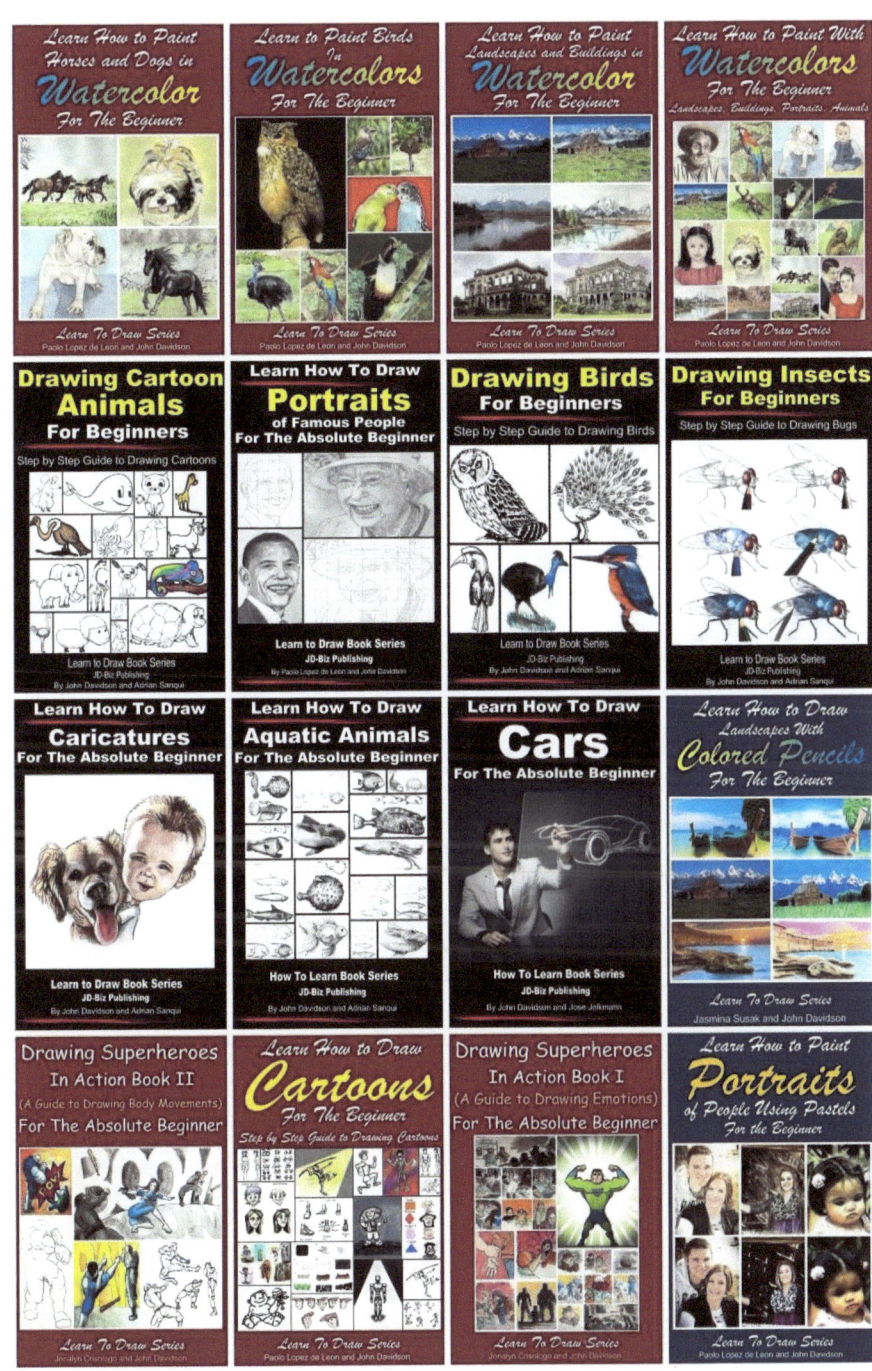

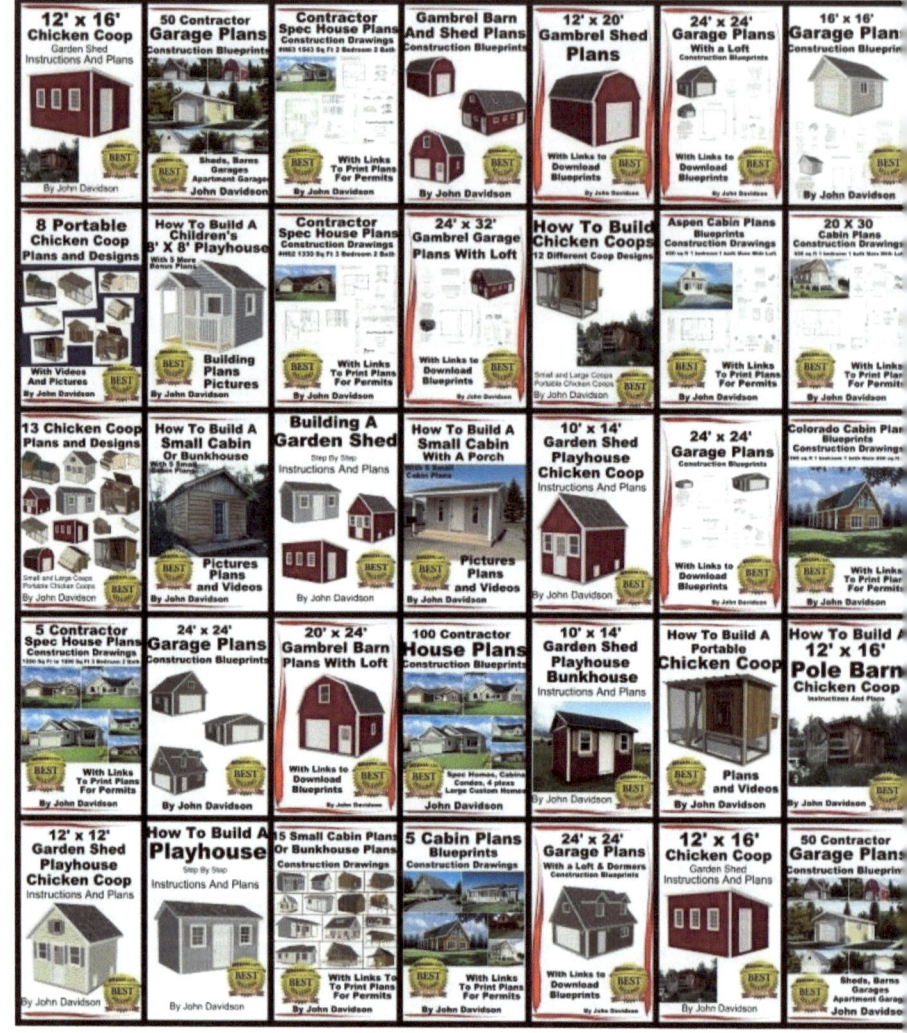

Entrepreneur Book Series

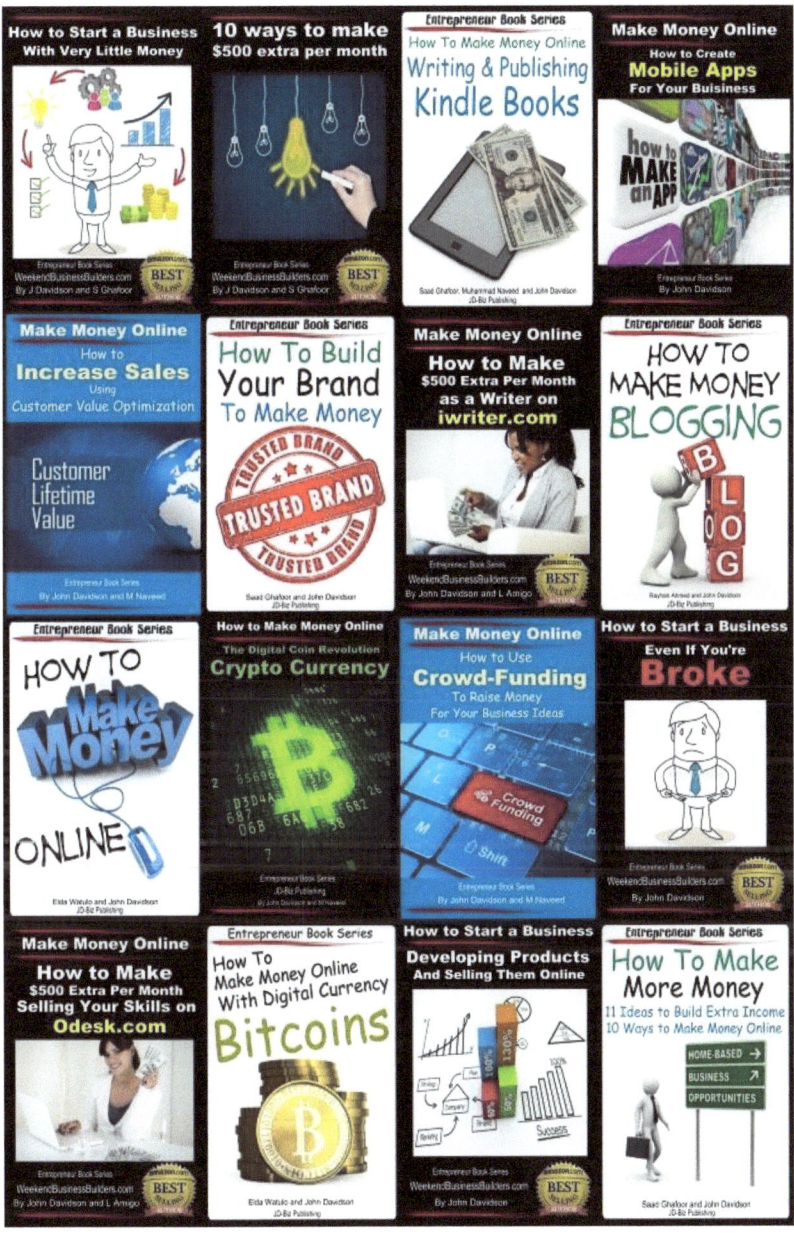

Our books are available at

1. Amazon.com
2. Barnes and Noble
3. Itunes
4. Kobo
5. Smashwords
6. Google Play Books

Download Free Books!

http://MendonCottageBooks.com

Publisher

JD-BIZ PUBLISHING

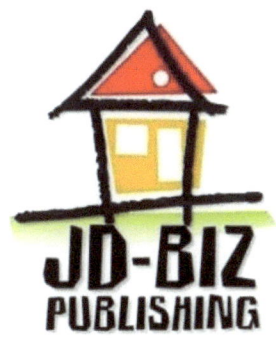

JD-Biz Corp

P O Box 374

Mendon, Utah 84325

http://www.jd-biz.com/

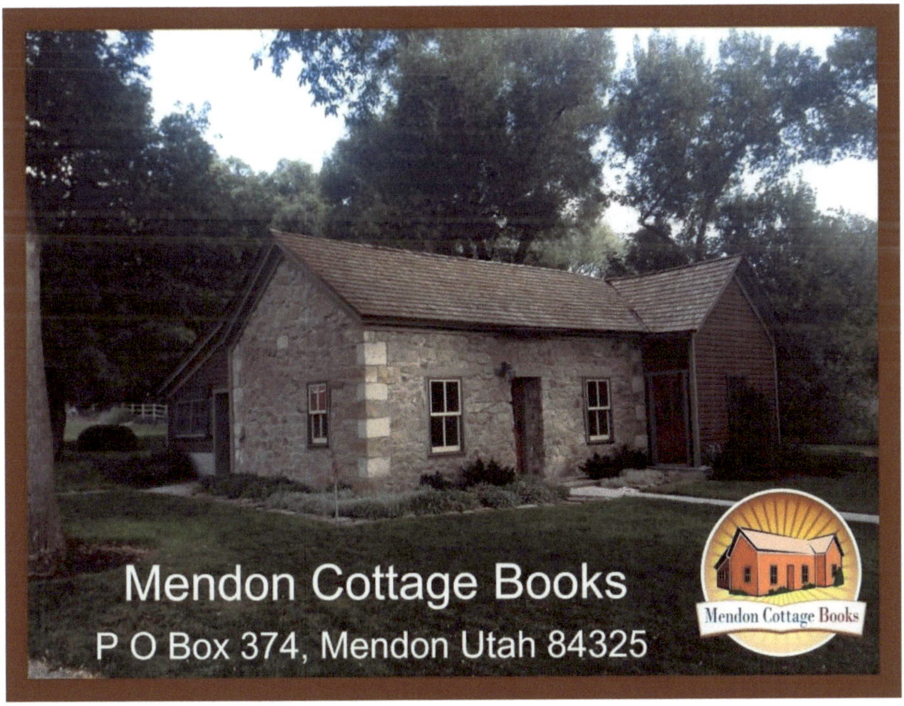

Mendon Cottage Books
P O Box 374, Mendon Utah 84325
Mendon Cottage Books

www.ingramcontent.com/pod-product-compliance
Lightning Source LLC
Chambersburg PA
CBHW050846290526
45792CB00002B/537